A Recipe For Health

A Recipe For Health

✦

The Truths You Should Know About Healthy Eating and Healthy Living.

Dr Ji Eng

iUniverse, Inc.

New York Lincoln Shanghai

A Recipe For Health
The Truths You Should Know About Healthy Eating and Healthy Living.

iUniverse books may be ordered through booksellers or by contacting:

iUniverse
2021 Pine Lake Road, Suite 100
Lincoln, NE 68512
www.iuniverse.com
1-800-Authors (1-800-288-4677)

This book is intended as a reference volume only, not as a medical manual. The ideas, procedures and suggestions contained herein are not intended as a substitute for consulting with your personal medical practitioner. Neither the publisher nor the author shall be responsible for any loss or damage allegedly arising from any information or suggestion in this book. Further, if you suspect that you have a medical problem, you should seek professional medical help.

ISBN-13: 978-0-595-36432-9 (pbk)
ISBN-13: 978-0-595-80864-9 (ebk)
ISBN-10: 0-595-36432-2 (pbk)
ISBN-10: 0-595-80864-6 (ebk)

Printed in the United States of America

Contents

1

INTRODUCTION

For years I have been treating patients with cardiovascular and chest diseases including patients with diabetes and cancer. I often wonder how patients, especially younger ones, develop these diseases. More often than not, following the conventional medical line, the answer is not clear. Obviously diet and lifestyle play an important role in the generation and persistence of many diseases.

With advances in medical knowledge and technology, presumably more and more people are aware of healthy lifestyle and healthy eating. More and more people are increasingly health conscious, exercising away in gyms and parks morning and evening. You would think that people are getting healthier and living longer.

Why is it then that sitting in my office, I see more and more patients with diabetes, heart disease and cancer? Could it be that what we believe to be a healthy lifestyle is wrong and that we are killing ourselves with all kinds of so-called healthy foods?

You would not think that big corporations would be out there to harm anybody, let alone produce 'poisons' that we daily put into our mouth. How wrong I was! The bottom line in food manufacturing, as is the case with organized medicine and pharmaceutical companies, is profit. You would think that if a product that is widely used is subsequently shown to be harmful, the relevant companies would withdraw it voluntarily. Instead, more often than not, these powerful companies would bring in their own paid 'experts' to counter the argument so that they can continue to market their products to produce increased profits. It is only when there is continued pressure from many quarters that something is withdrawn.

We all accept certain long believed concepts as gospel truths without looking into the background of the ideas. You would think that most beliefs that get passed from generation to generation are founded on solid research. You will be surprised to learn that many such concepts are based on very shaky researches which are subsequently proved wrong.

Unfortunately, if big business is involved, the subsequent research findings may be buried in some obscure corners that are not easily detected. Previously these are not disseminated at all, since almost all publications are supported by companies with vested interests which would more than likely suppress any adverse reports. However, with the advent of the Internet, all kinds of information can be made available to the interested reader. While many of these individuals and companies have their own agenda, there are enough conscientious people in the world who genuinely believe in benefiting mankind without resort to profiteering.

For years I have been advising my patients on various aspects of healthy living. Along the way I uncover many amazing facts which I feel would benefit more people than I am capable of coming into contact with. It is for this reason that I have decided to write this book. I hope it would form the backbone for the resurgence of healthy life-style which would promote better quality of life and longevity.

2

VESTED INTEREST

It seems clear to me that inevitably, whenever somebody or some company promotes a product, there is a vested interest involved. There must be a return to the investment that is made. Unfortunately and sadly, modern medical practice has also become more financially orientated.

Modern medicine is now a business. Individual doctors and hospital especially the private ones depend on profit generation in order to survive. The pressure for commercial success is so great that unless each individual keeps up with the tide, he is likely to get ostracized by colleagues and the public. In the background are the powerful pharmaceutical companies promoting all sorts of drugs for all types of diseases.

When doctors are in active practice, most of their so-called continuing medical education comes from pharmaceutical company representatives and sponsored talks. Sometimes, overseas speakers are flown in, at great expense (since many such speakers expect at least business class travels), to teach local doctors on new drugs that the companies have patented and thus have exclusive rights for sales.

These people are hardly likely to be very objective when talking about the drug or drugs the company is promoting. Furthermore, when medical representatives visit doctors at their clinics to promote drugs, they bring gifts to constantly remind doctors to prescribe their products. Doctors and their families are sometimes invited to seaside resorts for seminars at the expense of the drug companies.

Many doctors attend overseas conferences with their expenses totally covered by drug companies. Can you still genuinely believe that these doctors will not be influenced by such practices to prescribe drugs that are promoted? By the way, who is actually paying for these extravagances? Certainly not the drug companies since they are still making tons of money. Where does the money come from? It comes from consumers and patients, of course.

Thus, thousands of patients who pay for the drugs prescribed by the doctors indirectly also pay for those overseas holidays disguised as 'conferences'. From the companies' viewpoint, these are good investments since they still end up with hefty profits at the end of the financial year.

There is a more direct way that money is involved in modern medical practice. In many countries, doctors are not paid by the hospitals or health authorities. They are paid directly by the patients from the procedures that are performed. Herein lies the problem of objectivity.

For instance cardiologists are now actively promoting angioplasty for treatment of all forms of coronary artery disease, no matter whether the long-term results are good or otherwise. On the face of it, this is for the benefits of the patients who do not need to go for surgery, have only a 2mm scar on the groin instead of a few feet (some would even show pictures comparing the scars). However, to the cardiologist who is used to having big income from his practice and thus has heavy financial commitments, somebody has to pay the bills.

Thus, even when it is arguable whether angioplasty or surgery is superior for the overall wellbeing and also financial health of the patient (modern cardiology interventions are even more expensive than conventional surgery), cardiologists would come in favor of their own field. Since there are no checks and balances as the patients see the cardiologist alone all the way through, the avenue for abuse is ever present. Thus, the next time a doctor makes a decision regarding your health, think carefully whether it is in your best interest or in the interest of his own pocket.

3

DOCTORS AND HEALTH

Who is responsible for your health? This is an interesting question. Some people equate the availability of health care facilities and easy access to doctors as good signs of the health status of a country. They then go on with their unhealthy lifestyles, hoping that when they fall ill, their doctors will rescue them.

While it may be true that in many life-threatening situations doctors are able to help patients through their illnesses, in other, mainly chronic diseases, doctors are merely able to improve the patients to a small extent only. This patch-up job may or may not extend the longevity of the individual, although this may not be clear to the patients. Furthermore, many doctors are not very well informed about the preventive measures for diseases and nutrition. It is thus the responsibility of the patients themselves to learn as much as possible about the conditions concerned.

In the US, it is estimated that doctors caused 250,000 deaths a year from unnecessary surgery, medical and other errors, drug reactions and infections. This figure means that doctors are the third largest cause of death, after deaths from heart disease and cancer. There is evidence that the more doctors there are, the worse the number of iatrogenic (caused by treatment) diseases. This partly explains why in the US and other developed countries, despite huge expenditure on the national budget, the health of the nation as measured by various indexes is still way below the world league.

Perhaps you may think that governmental and regulatory bodies have a responsibility to look after your health. In fact, many doctors are more than willing to promote drugs and treatments that are approved by US regulatory authority as an assurance of safety. However, if you look at how the system works, then you may have your doubts about the effectiveness of this regulatory measure.

To be granted approval is a prerequisite for any drug and medical device before release to the general public. The process is very complex and entails huge expenses on the part of the drug companies concerned. Something like 240 million US dollars have to be spent to get a drug or medical device approved. Thus, only the financially strong multinational pharmaceutical companies can afford this kind of investment.

This partly explains why drug companies would only promote medications which they can pattern in order to recoup their investment. After all, they are in the business of making money. Of course, when they have to invest such huge sums of money on a product, they have to make absolutely certain that the approval is assured. Herein lie the potential dangers.

Drug companies apparently can manipulate the system with selective submission of studies to strengthen their arguments. Furthermore, there is strong financial and political pressure for well known companies to get swift approval. Apparently regulatory employees have strong links with drug companies. Many of these people, after their stints with the authority, seek employment with the giant pharmaceutical companies with big salaries and big bonuses. These people are not going to jeopardize their financial future with antagonism of the powerful drug companies.

Can we expect therefore that whatever decisions and judgments made by the regulatory authority represent the best interest of the consumers? Many instances in the past have clearly demonstrated that strong financial pressures resulted in many errors of judgment which subsequently caused the deaths of patients all round the world.

It is imperative that each one of us takes the responsibility to know as much as possible about healthy lifestyle and nutrition. By the time an illness has struck, it is probably too late to reverse the trend. It would be much better to prevent any illness from occurring in the first place with proper nutrition and other measures.

People who claim that nothing can be done to prevent illnesses are more likely than not ignorant of current thinking in many areas. Just because something is not accepted in conventional medical thinking does not mean there is no basis for the suggestion.

Thus, doctors and individuals have to be open minded about the world around them. We are talking about improving the quality of life and the quantity, if appropriate. The quality of life of someone who is ill in hospital is never going to be better than the same person while healthy and at liberty to choose whatever he wishes to pursue.

Many medical conditions, especially chronic ones, take years to develop. It is thus vital that each one of us takes the necessary steps towards achieving a healthy state through nutritional and other means as early as possible. Of course, you have to be armed with the necessary knowledge, and correct ones, if you are ever going to achieve the aim of a healthy body and a healthy mind. If you can lead a healthy life without visiting doctors or hospitals, then you should be a model for the rest of humanity.

4

DIET

There is no question in my mind that apart from the air we breathe in and the water we drink, food plays an important part in our health and wellbeing and therefore in many diseases. Even when food does not directly cause disease, it has a bearing on the progression of the disease and how our body can handle any insults to our cells. Even in the presence of invading organisms and viruses, our body's immune system may be able to overcome these without resort to drugs or surgery to regain our state of health.

A disease is the failure of our body to deal with unfavorable influences. Unfortunately there are numerous myths and misconceptions believed to be healthy practices which on more critical examination turn out to be the culprits in many conditions. Vested interests have prevented these to be widely disseminated.

The tragic consequence is our continued exposure to all kinds of poisons with the belief that they are actually healthy. Once the damage is done, it may be too late to reverse the changes. In many cases, once the tissues are damaged, they are totally irreversible.

5

FATS AND OILS

Of the three types of macronutrients in our food, fat is, I believe the most important for the maintenance of our health and wellbeing. There has also been the most misunderstanding, misquotation and mistakes in our appreciation of the importance of fats and oils.

Essentially fats and oils are made up of chains of carbon and hydrogen atoms bound together by covalent bonds. Each carbon atom is capable of forming four bonds with neighboring carbon and hydrogen atoms. When all four bonds are single bonds, the fat is saturated. When double bonds exist between the carbon atom backbone, the fat is unsaturated.

Monounsaturated fat has one double bond in its molecule while polyunsaturated fat has more than one double bonds. Saturated fat is stable and its straight molecules can be packed closely together to become solid fat at lower temperatures. On the other hand, the double bonds in polyunsaturated fat allow the molecules to bend and fold. In the natural form, they take on a cis formation. These configurations mean that the molecules cannot be packed tightly together.

Thus, polyunsaturated fat remains as oils in liquid form even at low temperatures. If you keep corn or sunflower oils with their high contents of polyunsaturated fats even in the freezer compartment of your refrigerator, they will not become solid. Contrast these with coconut oil, with its high content of saturated fat, which becomes solid in the refrigerator even outside the freezer compartment.

The unsaturated double bonds in the fatty acid chains, while conferring useful three-dimensional structures important for the formation of special channels and receptors, also mean that these molecules are more reactive. They can become easily oxidized and turn rancid. This happens in the presence of heat, light and oxygen. Once oxidized, they become catalysts in the generation of damaging chemicals. In our body, these generate free radicals which can lead to all kinds of diseases including heart disease, hypertension and even cancer.

Fats are vital components of our cells. In fact, the cell membrane consists mostly of a phospholipid bilayer. Fats give integrity and strength to the cell membrane. Our brain is 70% fat. Most of the fats are saturated fats in the form of triglycerides which are made up of three molecules of fatty acids attached to a glycerol. Our body is able to make saturated fat from sugar and protein. The long chain fatty acids are an efficient way to store energy.

Our body is also capable of converting stearic acid into monounsaturated oleic acid. However, our body is incapable of making many of the polyunsaturated fatty acids. These are therefore essential in our diet and are commonly known as essential fatty acids. Omega 3 fatty acids have three double bonds while omega 6 fatty acids have two double bonds. These are the commonest essential fatty acids.

Apart from the presence and number of double bonds, fats are also classified according to the number of carbon atoms and thus the length of the molecules. Short chain fatty acids have 4 to 6 carbon and are always saturated. The four carbon butyric acid and six carbon capric acid are both found in butter fat. Because of their short chains, they are easily absorbed and can be readily used by the liver for energy.

Median chain fatty acids have 8 to 12 carbon atoms. These are also saturated. They are also easily absorbed and utilized by the liver for energy. Long chain fatty acids have from 14 to 24 carbon atoms and they can be saturated, monounsaturated or polyunsaturated. The 16 carbon palmitoleic acid and 18 carbon stearic acid are both found in butter fat. They have strong antimicrobial properties, so have the short and medium chain fatty acids.

Most of the animal and vegetable sources of fats and oils have combinations of saturated and unsaturated fatty acids, short and long chains in combination with vitamins and other ingredients. It is useful to examine some of the more common types of fats and oils to clarify our knowledge and to make intelligent choices in our diet.

BUTTER

Butter contains a high concentration of short and median chain fatty acids and mostly saturated fatty acids. Butter is also rich in fat soluble vitamins A, D, E and K. There is also some cholesterol in butter, which gives butter a bad name. But as we shall see later, this really is not a problem.

BEEF AND LAMB TALLOW

These contain 50 to 55% saturated fat, 40% monounsaturated fat and less than 3% polyunsaturated fat. These are very heat stable and can be used for frying.

CHICKEN FAT

Chicken fat contains 31% saturated, 49% monounsaturated and 20% polyunsaturated fat. The higher content of polyunsaturated fat means lower stability and the polyunsaturated fats are more heat labile.

DUCK AND GOOSE FAT

These contain 35% saturated fat, 52% monounsaturated fat and 13% polyunsaturated fat. These are treated by the French as delicacies and are used for frying.

LARD

Lard has 40% saturated, 48 % monounsaturated and 12% polyunsaturated fat. It is a good source of vitamin D and is stable enough for frying.

The contents of animal fats vary according to the diet given to the animals. Thus, while animals roaming in the wild grassland have healthy proportion of saturated and polyunsaturated fatty acids, animals kept in enclosures and fed grain have poorer quality fats, vitamins, minerals and protein.

Since the half life of fat is 500 days, when we consume meats from animals fed unhealthy food and fats, we will also get the same unhealthy fats. This also applies to various chemicals, hormones and drugs including antibiotics which are introduced into our food chain via animal husbandry.

OLIVE OIL

Olive oil has more than 75% oleic acid, a monounsaturated fatty acid, 10% omega 6 polyunsaturated fatty acid and 2% omega 3. It is good for salad and medium temperature cooking.

SUNFLOWER, CORN, SOYA AND COTTONSEED OILS

These contain more than 50% omega 6 polyunsaturated fatty acids and minimal omega 3 fatty acid. Because of the high content of polyunsaturated fatty acids, these oils should never be heated as in frying or baking.

CANOLA OIL

Canola oil contains 57% oleic acid, 23% omega 6 and 10-15% omega 3 fatty acid. It is made from rape seed which belongs to the mustard family. Canola stands for Canadian oil which the industry believed is a better term than rape seed oil. It is marketed as a good oil due to its high omega 3 content. Unfortunately, the processing of canola oil and other seed derived oils have so damaged the fatty acids that they are relatively poisonous to the body.

PEANUT OIL

This has 48% monounsaturated oleic acid, 18% saturated fat and 34% omega 6 polyunsaturated fatty acid.

SESAME OIL

Sesame oil contains 42% oleic acid, 15% saturated fat and 43% omega 6 polyunsaturated fatty acid.

FLAX SEED OIL

This oil has a high content of omega 3 polyunsaturated fatty acid (57%), 18% oleic acid, 16% omega 6 fatty acid and 9% saturated fat.

COCONUT OIL

Coconut oil contains a high percentage of saturated fat, 86.5% with 5.8% monounsaturated and 1.8% polyunsaturated fatty acids. Because of this, coconut oil is very stable and is considered by some to be the healthiest oil on earth.

PALM OIL

Palm oil contains 37% monounsaturated fatty acids, 49.3% saturated fatty acids and 9.3% polyunsaturated fatty acids.

PROBLEMS WITH VEGETABLE OILS

It looks at first sight that many vegetable oils have high levels of the so-called essential fatty acids, omega 3 and omega 6, and are thus marketed as healthy oils to be used in our diet. There has to be a fine balance between omega 6 and omega 3 since omega 6 tend to increase the production of pro-inflammatory prostaglandins while omega 3 tend to be the reverse. A healthy ratio of omega 6 to omega 3 may be 4:1. Most of our vegetable oils contain an excess of omega 6 which is detrimental to our health.

On deeper analysis however, the detrimental effects of processed vegetable oils are much more profound than the ratio of omega 6 to omega 3. These polyunsaturated fatty acids, by the presence of the double bonds in their molecules, are easily damaged. They become oxidized and turn rancid.

The damage occurs in the presence of heat, light and oxygen. Thus, unless careful measures are taken during the extraction and processing of these vegetable oils, the end products contain a high percentage of damaged fatty acids which are detrimental to our body. This is what happens in the large scale industrial processing of soybean, sunflower, corn, canola and peanut oils.

The processing involves also using deodorizing and bleaching agents which may remain in small amounts in the finished products. Contrast this to the gentle, cold compression of virgin olive oil. Thus, virgin olive oil is truly virgin in preserving the natural, undamaged oleic and polyunsaturated fatty acids. However, with high heat, even this can be damaged.

Since modern day industrial processing of seed oil damages polyunsaturated fatty acids, the higher the content of polyunsaturated fatty acids, the greater the damage in the finished products. These are what the edible oil industry wants to get everyone to use instead of the traditional oils including animal fats and tropical oils.

Even when polyunsaturated fatty acids are not damaged, they should never be used in high temperature cooking including frying, baking and deep frying. Furthermore, repeated heating damages the oils even more. Modern fast food restaurants use a lot of vegetable oils in their cooking. Is it any wonder that we are now faced with numerous problems and diseases which can be traced directly or indirectly to the consumption of processed, damaged vegetable oils?

This sorry state of affairs has prevailed partly due to the ingenuity of man in finding a solution to the problem of surplus, excess vegetable seed oil. In the nineteenth century, seed oils including soybean oil were used in paints. Some clever chemist then invented a method to make cheaper paint from petroleum waste products. The seed oil industry was left with excess vegetable oils with no avenues for disposal.

At the time, the majority of the population was consuming large quantities of animal fats. Early in the 1950's Ancel Keys suggested, on his observation of arterial disease, that saturated fat and cholesterol were the cause of heart disease. Substituting saturated animal fat with vegetable oils appeared to reduce the cholesterol level and thus arterial disease. The seed oil industry thus seized on this preliminary observation to promote their oils as heart healthy. Even though subsequently these were found to be contentious, the industry has become so powerful and so established that it is well nigh impossible to say otherwise.

MARGARINE

The same human ingenuity allowed chemists to convert vegetable oil into margarine which was marketed as a cheap, supposedly healthy alternative to butter. In the 1930's and during the second world war, food was scarce and butter was expensive. Some clever chemists worked out that the cheap vegetable oil could be transformed into imitation butter and this was then marketed as heart friendly. Unfortunately, this is a purely man made stuff not found in nature. Our body is thus exposed to another powerful toxin with undesirable side effects.

As discussed previously, polyunsaturated vegetable oils would remain liquid even at low temperatures due to the molecular three dimensional structures. To transform this liquid oil into solid margarine, the oil has to be treated with hydrogen in high pressures and temperatures and in the presence of metallic catalysts including cobalt, nickel and aluminium. The folded molecule of the polyunsaturated fatty acid then become straightened so that they can be tightly packed together to form solid margarine. Thus the natural cis fatty acid becomes trans fatty acid. This is the process of hydrogenation.

Hydrogenated or partially hydrogenated vegetable oils are widely used in the food industry, especially baking, since they appear to improve the shelf life of the foods. Unfortunately, the damaged polyunsaturated fatty acids, or trans fatty acids, are extremely injurious to our cells.

I believe that whatever confusion remains regarding animal fats or vegetable oils, everyone has to agree that poisons are not good to our body. Since hydrogenated oils and trans fatty acids are solely man made and not found in nature, our body would not have evolved to deal with this kind of damaged chemicals without side effects. In fact, this fat would still be incorporated into our cell membranes resulting in leaky cells unable to hold onto electrolytes and water, and nonfunctioning receptors.

This may be the basis of many of our present day diseases, including diabetes, heart disease and cancer. As the half life of fat in our body is five hundred days, it takes years for us to get rib of all these poisons even if we were able to stop consuming them straight away. Unfortunately, these damaged oils are so prevailing in all sorts of manufactured foods, most of which do not carry this information in their labels, it is almost impossible to avoid them unless we are extremely careful.

The knowledge that trans fats are damaging to our body and our heart has been published over forty years ago. Unfortunately, big business and other vested interests have curtailed the circulation of this damaging information. Merely labeling the trans fat content of food items was too strong for the food industry which has resisted despite strong arguments from informed lipid researches. They are more than happy to label their content of polyunsaturated fatty acids and zero cholesterol to attract business.

After years of lobbying, the US Congress finally accepted that food labels should carry the content of trans fat so that consumers can make a choice. Since there are no benefits from trans fats which are damaging to the body, this step may have serious implications for the industry. Naturally big business managed to postpone the date for the start of this step to 2006. In the meantime, consumers are still exposed to dangerous levels of damaging fats without the facility to identify it. However, hydrogenated or partially hydrogenated fats are sometimes labeled. These should be avoided at all costs.

RECYCLING GONE CRAZY

While big businesses and pharmaceutical companies are out to maximize their profits by whatever means or manipulations at their disposal, including influencing political parties and government agencies, the average trader is also in the market trying to make more money by increasing their profit margin. Competition obviously plays a part in driving prices down. Thus, the more intangible way would be to reduce the cost of production. In the food industry, the use of recycled oil is one such way to maximize profits.

Until a few months ago, I was ignorant of the usage of recycled oil in the food industry, especially the hawkers. It was a patient who told me of a shop whose sole business is to supply recycled oil to the food industry. We all know that hawkers who sell deep fried food used the same pot of oil again and again, at least until the end of the trading day.

What I did not know was that the original oil used by these traders is recycled from big restaurants which use a lot of oil in their food preparation. In fact, even the containers for the oil may be recycled items. While saving the environment, we pour these poisons back into our stomach and wonder why people get sick. Apparently this is common knowledge among hawkers and restauranters.

The common people probably do not appreciate the dangers this practice poses, since 'everybody is doing it'. The tragedy is that the original polyunsaturated vegetable oils are already damaged even before the first generation user started using it. The recycled stuff is obviously more damaged and thus more poisoinous.

A NEW WAY OF COOKING

Since even the heat stable butter and tropical oils can be damaged when heated to extremes of temperatures, there is a need for change in our philosophy and practice of cooking. Thus, deep frying is never a good way to cook.

Traditionally people, especially the Chinese, heat the oil first to high temperatures, and then add in the ingredients in stages. The temperatures achieved in a hot wok can be very high. However, instead of oil, if we were to start with water, then the temperature cannot go beyond 100 degrees Centigrade, the boiling point of water, provided there is water left to boil.

Hence if meat or vegetables are added before the water dries up, then the temperature would be more moderate that if cooking oils were used initially. At the end of this, when the heating has been stopped, some oils can be added if desired. In this case, coconut oil or even olive oil can be added with assurance that they will not be damaged by high heat.

Cooking is a natural part of the daily activity in most cultures. Many people, especially strict vegetarians, advocate salad and uncooked foods. While some food items are easily handled by out digestive system even in the raw state, many others need to be cooked before our body can digest the ingredients. Furthermore, cooking destroys bacteria and other harmful elements in our foods. Thus, intelligent cooking is vital to produce the best tasting and healthiest food for the nourishment of our body.

COCONUT OIL—THE HEALTHIEST OIL ON EARTH

Persistent propaganda by the American edible oil industry has permeated even the remotest corners of the earth so that everybody believes that coconut oil is bad for health and bad for cholesterol. However, the original research on the effect of coconut oil on cholesterol levels in experimental animals apparently made use of damaged, hydrogenated coconut oil. When badly treated, even the best oils can be damaged to become poisonous to our body.

Coconut oil has a high content of saturated fatty acid, about 90%, which is why it is heat stable. In fact, since coconuts are daily exposed to high temperatures in nature, the oil has to be stable. Otherwise, all the coconut trees would have died off in the tropical heat.

The remarkable thing about the saturated fat in coconut is the high content of medium chain fatty acid, of which the most abundant is lauric acid, forming about 60%. These medium chain fatty acids have remarkable properties, all of which contribute to our wellbeing.

This is why coconut oil has been used in some traditional cultures for thousands of years. Incidentally, mother's breast milk also contains a high concentration of median chain fatty acids. These are important for the nourishment and development of the baby.

The medium chain fatty acids and triglycerides are handled differently by our digestive tract. They can be absorbed directly into our intestinal blood stream without emulsification and other digestive processes. After absorption, they are delivered to the liver. These oils can get into the mitochondria and be utilized for energy much more easily than the longer chain fatty acids. Thus, it is a good source of energy for the body, which explains why medium chain fatty acids are widely used in intravenous nutritional preparations for intensive care unit patients requiring nutritional support.

These medium chain fatty acids especially lauric acid but also caprylic acid, caproic acid and capric acid, have remarkable healing properties. These enhance our immune system. In the laboratory, these fatty acids have been shown to have antibacterial, antiviral and antifungal properties.

These have been shown to be beneficial to our digestive health and may be beneficial in patients with diseases of the digestive system including Crohn's disease and irritable bowel syndrome.

Coconut oil improves thyroid function more by uncoupling the suppressant effect of polyunsaturated fats rather than the actual stimulation of the thyroid gland. This may be one reason why coconut oil can be part of the program for weight loss. Preliminary studies in patients with HIV and AIDS in the Philippines have shown some encouraging results in reducing the viral load and also improving the nutrition of these patients.

Since coconut oil is so good, every part of the edible coconut is potentially health promoting. Coconut water was good enough to be infused directly into the blood stream as a fluid replacement during the war when the supply of intravenous fluids ran out. Young coconut meat is very refreshing. Coconut milk can be used in coffee, cooking and in baking. It is a great shame that we are foregoing something so easily available in our doorsteps in favor of man-made margarine and hydrogenated oils, greatly damaging our health in the process. This goes to show how powerful a tool propaganda and slick marketing can do.

6

CHOLESTEROL

By now, everybody knows about cholesterol, about how damaging cholesterol in the diet is and everybody is on low-fat, low cholesterol, 'heart-friendly' diet. You would think that something as profound as cholesterol and its supposed ill effects have been thoroughly researched beyond reasonable doubt and the conclusion cast in stones. Why would doctors, especially cardiologists, keep harping on about high cholesterol being the cause of heart disease and keep measuring cholesterol levels in your blood and prescribing expensive drugs to millions of patients worldwide? However, a critical analysis of the available evidence casts considerable doubt on any of these exertions.

Cholesterol is a high molecular weight alcohol made in large quantities by all the cells in the body, especially the liver. It is an essential component of the cell membrane and is present in high concentration in the brain. Together with saturated fats, cholesterol in the cell membrane gives the cell stiffness and stability.

Cholesterol is a precursor for corticosteroid and sex hormones like testosterone, estrogen and progesterone and also for vitamin D. Bile salts are made from cholesterol. Cholesterol acts as an antioxidant. It is needed for the proper functioning of serotonin receptors in the brain. Cholesterol is also important for the proper functioning of the intestinal wall.

How would something as important for the body as cholesterol become the cause of heart disease? How would cholesterol become bad when it is associated with low density lipoprotein (LDL) and good if associated with high density lipoprotein (HDL)? Is cholesterol suffering from 'guilty by association' or are we barking up the wrong tree?

Cholesterol and saturated fat were implicated as a causative agent in coronary artery disease when the lipid hypothesis was proposed in the 1953 by Ancel Keys in his 'Seven Countries Study'. In 1954 a Russian researcher, David Kritchevsky published a paper describing the effects of feeding cholesterol to rabbits which caused the formation of atheromas.

Observations on young American soldiers killed in action in Korea appeared to show the presence of atheroma even in soldiers in their twenties. The presence of cholesterol in the atheromas does not necessarily mean that cholesterol itself is the cause of arterial disease. In fact, some researchers believe that cholesterol is the healing substance recruited into the atheroma when the damage has already occurred.

Since cholesterol has an antioxidant function, this may be a manifestation of the healing property of cholesterol. Furthermore, there is a higher proportion of unsaturated fatty acid, especially polyunsaturated fatty acid in the atheromatous plaques. Granted that cholesterol itself can be damaged and can then cause tissue damage.

Many epidemiological studies have been carried out to find a link between the consumption of cholesterol in the diet and the incidence of heart disease. The best known of these is probably the Framingham Heart Study started in 1948 and is still continuing. After twenty two years of study, the researchers concluded that there was no suggestion of any relation between diet and the subsequent development of coronary heart disease.

Interventional study like the Multiple Risk Factor Interventional Trial did not show a beneficial effect on coronary artery disease or total mortality. A review of twenty six studies in 1992 concluded that lowering cholesterol did not reduce mortality and was unlikely to prevent coronary heart disease.

Coronary artery disease was virtually unknown in the earliest decades of the twentieth century. In fact, when an American physician introduced the electro-cardiograph machine invented in Germany into his American hospital, he was advised to find something more useful to do, since coronary heart disease, which this machine was designed to pick up, was so rare. Studies on the American diet in those days showed that the typical diet consisted of a large proportion of saturated fats and cholesterol.

From the 1950's to the present time, coronary artery disease has become the leading cause of death in most developed and many developing countries. This has occurred despite the fact that the consumption of cholesterol and saturated fats has decreased, probably from widespread misinformation of the supposed risks of these substances in our diet.

If cholesterol and saturated fats were the culprits, then reducing the intake in our diet surely would reduce our risks of getting heart disease. However, the trend seems to be the reverse. Despite widespread knowledge about the risks of high cholesterol and saturated fats, the prevalence of heart disease has increased in most countries.

If it is not cholesterol and saturated fats that cause heart disease, then what is the cause? There is considerable evidence that the vegetable cooking oils, hydrogenated and partially hydrogenated oils, and margarine are the real culprits that not only cause heart disease but also cancer and diabetes.

As explained in the previous chapter, these were introduced in the 1950's as replacements for animal fats, butter and tropical oils and very strongly promoted by the edible oil industry as healthier alternatives. Thus, the consumption has shot up by leaps and bounds. Every housewife knows about the 'heart-friendly' margarine and butter has become taboo.

If you plot the trend in the consumption of margarine, it parallels the increase in heart disease, and also cancer, whereas that of cholesterol and saturated fats was decreasing. Thus, if anything, it is the margarine and hydrogenated vegetable oils that are causing the epidemic of heart disease and cancer, rather than cholesterol and saturated fats.

Why is it then that this kind of knowledge is not widely disseminated for the good of the public? How is it that despite lack of concrete evidence of cholesterol being the cause of heart disease, the public is so aware of the risks of high cholesterol and saturated fats? I suppose it boils down to propaganda and vested interests.

It is estimated that the American edible oil industry is a multibillion enterprise involving thousands of individuals from farmers to oil processors and distributors. The biggest of them, the soybean oil producers, has an annual turnover of about seven billion dollars. Such powerful players can influence many things by their lobbying and slick marketing. They were largely responsible for claiming that tropical oils were damaging to the heart and should be avoided like the plague. With such huge financial power, they were able to influence various bodies including the medical profession and even governmental policy makers to issue guidelines favorable to their industry.

Funding for university research projects is based on the favorable results that these are expected to produce for the industry. Even professional bodies and scientific journals are not immune to this pressure. Thus a researcher who proposes to study the detrimental aspects of the vegetable oils might have considerable difficulty getting the necessary funding for the project. Even when the studies are done independently to show adverse results, these may not get published in reputable journals which rely on advertising revenues for their survival.

7

SUGAR AND CARBOHYDRATE

The misconception about fat and cholesterol had led to a major shift of our diet from high fat diet to high carbohydrate diet, with dire consequences. Dietitians and nutritionists, even doctors, advise patients, especially patients with diabetes, to cut down on sugar or avoid sugar. They are then advised to cut down on fats, and by extension, meat and animal products for fear of getting heart disease, cancer and all kinds of other diseases.

In fact, the food pyramid as advocated by the American Dietectic Association, the American Diabetic Association, the American Heart Association etc has carbohydrate as the base. Patients are advised to eat lots of complex carbohydrates while avoiding sugar, fats, cholesterol and thus high cholesterol meats.

Whatever sugars and carbohydrates we consume end up as simple sugars after digestion in our stomach and intestine before these can be absorbed into our blood stream. Simple sugars are glucose, fructose, galactose etc whereas complex carbohydrates contain long chains of these simple sugars which are eventually broken down into simple sugars. Thus when we consume glucose, it can directly be absorbed without enzymatic action in our digestive tract.

However, starch, which is a long chain of glucose, takes time to digest and thus would not lead to high blood glucose level immediately. The body, on the other hand, is unable to distinguish the glucose that comes from simple, white refined sugar from glucose that comes from complex carbohydrate like that found in whole-meal or brown bread.

While avoiding sugars, if we consume large amounts of complex carbohydrate, the end result, that is the amount of simple sugars that get into our blood stream, is the same except the time of arrival is different. A high glucose load two hours after eating is going to have the same detrimental effects as the same load immediately after ingestion. A misunderstanding of this simple concept has resulted in wrong advice being given to patients, especially those with diabetes, with the result that they are put on larger and larger doses of drugs or insulin but their control is still less than ideal.

Our body cells make use of simple sugars like glucose for energy. It used to be believed that the brain is dependent on the availability of glucose for proper function. However, it is now believe that even the brain can make use of fats, and their breakdown products, ketone bodies, for energy.

The preferred fuel for heart muscle cells appears to be fatty acids. Glucose does make a readily available source of energy for body cells. Unfortunately, our body is unable to store large amount of glucose. There is a small amount stored as glycogen in the liver and muscle. The excess is converted to fat for long term storage, and there is no limit for this.

Too much sugar is no good for anybody. I don't think that anybody would dispute this. However, our body is able to control the level of glucose in our blood to maintain it at a good level, neither too high nor too low. It does this via the action of insulin. In response to high glucose level in the blood, the pancreas secretes insulin which acts on liver and other cells in our body to take up glucose for energy production or storage.

On the other hand, if for any reason the glucose level is too low, our body produces glucagon which tends to increase the glucose level by the liver cells releasing glucose from glycogen and protein by a process called gluconeogenesis. If all that the hormone insulin can do is to regulate the blood glucose level, then perhaps it is not too detrimental to have a higher level. New evidence has emerged that insulin has wide ranging metabolic, physiological and pathological effects.

Insulin is necessary for the conversion of glucose to fat. This storage hormone is essential for our body fat cells to accumulate fat. This partly explains why people get fat from eating high carbohydrate diet and not from eating low carbohydrate high fat diet since insulin has to be stimulated for a person to get fat. Diets such as the Atkins, South Beach, Zone and high protein diets are based on their effects on insulin.

Insulin in excess, hyperinsulinemia, occurs when excessive sugar is taken in our diet. Excessive insulin leads to the production of pro-inflammatory prostaglandins which act on all cells and tissues in our body. Total body inflammatory changes occur, resulting in high blood pressure, heart disease, arthritis, inflammatory bowel disease, cancer and other degenerative diseases. It probably has a bearing on aging. In the case of coronary artery disease, there is evidence that rather than cholesterol, C-reactive protein, which is a measure of the body's inflammation, is a more accurate predictor.

Hyperinsulinemia, or excessive insulin, is probably present in a large percentage of the population in most developed or developing countries. The end of the spectrum represents people with diabetes. It is now known that most people with adult onset diabetes or type II diabetes have high levels of insulin in their blood early in the course of their condition.

In fact, they have probably been exposed to high levels of insulin for years before they are found to be diabetic. Glucose levels form a continuous spectrum depending on the diet and physical activity. The cut off point for diabetes is arbitrarily determined. Thus, a difference of a minimal percentage may put somebody into a diabetic group, or out of it, depending on which direction is taken.

It is more relevant to talk about the control of glucose rather than to label patients into groups based on a sampling on the continuous scale of blood glucose. It is believed that hyperinsulinemia affects more than 50% of the American population. These are the overweight and obese individuals who are heading down the slope to the snare of diabetes unless some drastic changes are made to their diet.

Actually, glucose control is a relatively simple measure, if you have the right kind of advice and knowledge. Instead of relying on medications and insulin injection, the right amount of blood glucose can be achieved by modifying the diet. All that it necessary is a glucometer which quickly and simply measures the glucose in the blood from a drop of your blood.

Now when a high level of blood glucose is obtained, then it can only mean that there has been too much sugar and carbohydrate in the diet. You would not get excessive glucose level from the glucose generated by your own body. Thus, reducing the carbohydrate in the diet is the therapeutic maneuver that will reduce and eventually cure you of your diabetes, if you are diligent enough.

If you reduce your carbohydrate intake to such an extent that your blood glucose level remains below the diabetic level, then there is no need for medications and insulin injections which merely act to bring down the excessive glucose derived from the food. Since we can survive on very little or no carbohydrate in our diet, this surely is a more logical approach to the management of diabetes, which after all is the end of a spectrum of glucose levels in the blood, rather than relying on pharmaceuticals and insulin injections, all of which carry potentially damaging side effects.

The glycemic index is an indication of how much a food will raise blood glucose level. However, this is only a rough guide since each person's metabolism is different depending on digestion, absorption and rate of utilization. It is more important to determine, for each individual, the effect of each food on the blood glucose level so that fine tuning can be made.

If we reduce the amount of carbohydrate in our diet, then we will have to increase the amount of the other two macronutrients, fat and protein. Bearing in mind from our previous discussion on fats and oils, only the natural, undamaged fats and oils are useful and essential to our cells. As to proteins, we need the essential amino acids for cellular repair and regeneration of wear and tear.

There is evidence that high protein diet has a cellular protective effect independent of the dietary fat. Isomeric substitution of protein for carbohydrate can lead to a reduction of low density lipoprotein cholesterol and triglyceride, and an increase in high density lipoprotein. It may result in improved blood pressure and weight reduction. This can be explained by the reduction in insulin action. Even if some of the protein is converted to glucose by the liver, the level is unlikely to rival that achieved from eating high carbohydrate diet.

THE DAMAGING EFFECTS OF SUGAR

In the laboratory, when glucose is added to white blood cells, the phagocytic activity of the white blood cells is suppressed. This contributes to a reduction in the body's defence against bacterial infection. Sugar can suppress the immune system. Sugar can cause kidney damage by the process of glycosylation of the kidney filtering membrane.

Sugar contributes to peptic ulcers, Crohn's disease, ulcerative colitis, arthritis, asthma, gallstones, yeast infections, tooth decay and periodontal disease. Osteoporosis, varicose veins, obesity, migraine, cataracts, emphysema, atherosclerosis, increase in free radicals in the blood streams are all the potential side effects of excessive sugar consumption.

Sugar can decrease growth hormone and thus lead to aging. Sugar can impair the structure of DNA and thus contributes to the development of cancer. Sugar can cause drowsiness and decreased activity in children. Sugar can also cause hyperactivity, anxiety, difficulty in concentration and crankiness in children.

With such wide ranging damaging effects, we should drastically reduce our intake of sugar, or better still, eliminate it altogether. This is particularly important in patients who are already diabetic. When they do this however, they have to reduce the amount of diabetic medications or insulin injection. Otherwise, hypoglycemia may ensue. This is potentially life threatening.

Knowing the potential problems with insulin, it is illogical to commence patients on insulin early in the course of diabetic management, as still practiced by some doctors. This is especially so in many patients whose insulin levels, instead of being low, are elevated. Increasing hyperinsulinemia by insulin injection may compound the damaging effects of insulin.

INSULIN RESISTANCE AND HYPERINSULINEMIA

What causes excessive insulin levels in the blood? While too much stimulation from excessive sugar and carbohydrate intake in the diet obviously can play a part, there is a more fundamental process known as insulin resistance. This means that cells are not responsive to insulin in the blood. Thus, the pancreas has to secrete higher levels of insulin in order to achieve a reduction in blood glucose level.

People who are overweight and obese are known to be insulin resistant and require higher insulin levels, i.e. hyperinsulinemia. This can be reduced by weight reduction. People who are able to bring down their weight improve their diabetic control, blood pressure control and achieve a more favorable lipid profile.

There may be a molecular explanation for the development of insulin resistance and hyperinsulinemia. Insulin receptors on the cell membrane are composed of specific polyunsaturated fatty acids, proteins and carbohydrates with precise three dimensional configuration so that insulin molecules can interact to bring about the desired effects. The glucose transporters are then activated. These then transport the glucose into the cytoplasm and mitochondria where glucose is burnt for energy generation.

The glucose transporters are also dependent on the essential fatty acids with natural, undamaged configuration for proper function. If instead of the natural essential fatty acids, there is abundant damaged fatty acids like trans fat, then this is incorporated into the insulin receptors and glucose transporters, with the results that there are less responsive to insulin.

In order to overcome this, our body secretes more insulin. Since hyperinsulinemia has wide ranging pro-inflammatory effects on the other metabolic pathways, this leads to detrimental changes in our body. This may be the explanation why there is such widespread occurrence of mainly degenerative diseases not only with diabetes and its associated diseases but also other diseases like arthritis, inflammatory bowel disease and even cancer.

THE HEALING PROPERTIES OF NATURAL SUGARS

When we talk about the damaging effects of sugars, we refer to too much refined sugars with high contents of glucose. Too much fructose found in fruits is also damaging to the body. However, there are simple, natural sugars which are beneficial to our health. The study of these beneficial effects of simple sugars is called glycobiology.

Recent studies have shown that apart from glucose and galactose, there are six other essential sugars which are extremely important for our health. These are mannose, fucose, xylose, N-acetylglucosamine, N-acetylgalactosamine and N-acetylneuraminic acid. These eight essential sugars form a matrix surrounding the cells. They also combine with proteins and lipids on the surface of the cells and also within the cells. They are important for intercellular communication. Deficiency in one or more of these simple sugars may result in one of the many degenerative diseases encountered today.

These glyconutrients are found in nature. Unfortunately, intensive agricultural methods and food processing have resulted in considerable shortage of the simple sugars. Our body can manufacture the simple sugars from glucose. Unfortunately, stress, damaged fats and oils, and countless toxins have diminished our body's ability to provide adequately for these essential sugars. Eating fruits, vegetables and other sources of the sugars, for instance, kelp, eggs, shark and beef cartilage can supplement our needs for these sugars.

Some of these simple, essential sugars have, by themselves, good healing properties. Mannose, for instance is a simple sugar which has been found to be very effective in treating bladder and urinary tract infection. More than 90% of cases of urinary tract infection are caused by the bacteria E. Coli. Mannose, which is not broken down by our body, is secreted by the kidney. It binds to the bacteria thus preventing them from anchoring to the lining of the urinary tract, allowing the urine to flush out the infection. This is the active ingredient in cranberry juice which has been used for eliminating urinary tract infection especially in women, for years.

Aloe vera is a very rich source of mannose. This probably accounts for the great healing power of aloe vera juice and extract which have been used very effectively for healing of skin ulcers and other conditions. It probably helps in patients with cancers by improving their general wellbeing and their ability to undergo chemotherapy and other forms of treatment.

Xylitol is another sugar which has been found very useful in reducing ear and sinus infection. This sugar is found in plums and can be made from wood and wheat grass. Xylitol nasal spray effectively eliminate nasal and sinus infections. Xylitol has also been found very effective in reducing tooth decay. It inhibits Streptococcus mutants which is the bacterium that causes cavities. Xylitol chewing gum can be effective in restoring dental health.

Policosanol can be extracted from sugar cane. It has the ability to reduce cholesterol and triglyceride levels even more effectively than statin drugs without the side effects associated with these drugs. It was also found to reduce blood pressure, whereas statin drugs did not.

8

WATER

How many times have you experienced, turning on the tap only to find brown water flowing out? Even when the water is crystal clear, can we assume that it is safe to drink? Incidentally, if you own a filter, just look at the dirt that can collect on the filter cartridge after a short period of usage. Boiling the water may sterilize the water but this is not going to remove all the potential contaminants in the water.

Water is an important constituent of our body, forming 75 to 80% of our body weight. Our blood is more than 90% water. Life is not possible without water. Unfortunately, our sources of water have been contaminated by industrial and agricultural wastes.

Such water is taken from rivers and lakes, pumped to water treatment plants where it is filtered through sand and activated carbon, chlorinated and fluoridated and pH adjusted. After treatment, the water is pumped to a high rise reservoir to be distributed to consumers. This water has to travel via miles of water mains, some of which are clogged up through years of exposure to hard water.

Even in the 1960's, more than 2500 compounds were found in drinking water. Over the years, more and more chemicals have been manufactured and discharged eventually into our water sources. Most of these chemicals have potentials to do harm to our body.

ACID BASE BALANCE

To understand the importance of drinking healthy water, we need to have some knowledge of the acid-alkaline status of our body. Acidity is measured using pH scale of 0 to 14. 7 is exactly neutral. Less than 7 is acidic and more than 7, alkaline. Our body is maintained at a narrow pH range of 7.35 to 7.45, in an alkaline environment.

Most of our metabolic processes produce acids which are then neutralised. The waste is then removed from our body via the lungs or the urine. Maintaining a healthy alkaline range is important since our cells can only function well within this range. Too acid an environment is detrimental to the enzymes in our cells.

One theory of aging maintains that aging results from the accumulation of too much acidic waste products in our body. In 1931, Dr Otto Warburg was awarded the Nobel prize for demonstrating that the primary cause of cancer was the acidic environment generated via the fermentation of sugar in the absence of oxygen.

Patients with high blood pressure, gout, atherosclerosis and other degenerative diseases have abnormal build up of acidic waste in the body. Uric acid, however, is soluble in alkaline water. The formation of kidney stones and arthritis also results from an acid environment.

WATER PURIFICATION

From the above discussion, it may be assumed that the purer the water, the healthy it is for drinking. Thus, is distilled water, which is the purest form of water, the healthiest water for daily consumption? Apparently not.

Distilled water, as well as water from reverse osmosis, is devoid of useful minerals and electrolytes. Furthermore, these types of purified water are very active in absorbing substances from the environment. Thus, carbon dioxide easily dissolves in distilled water. As a result, the pH of distilled water is 4.5 and that of reverse osmosis water, 5. These acidic forms of water, taken for long period, may be detrimental to our health in generating a more acidic environment in our body, which already is full of all kinds of acids.

Purified water is beneficial when somebody is seeking to detoxify the body for a short period of perhaps a few weeks. Long term consumption of these relatively soft water leads to spill over of electrolytes and minerals, the result of which may be increased risk of osteoporosis, osteoarthritis, high blood pressure and coronary artery disease.

THE DETRIMENTAL EFFECTS OF CARBONATED SODA

All carbonated soda drinks which are so popular in the present culture are made from purified water. Most of these contain high concentration of sugars. In addition, the addition of carbon dioxide to make it gassy means that the pH of these drinks are in the region of 2.5. This level of acidity is clearly harmful to our body.

The high consumption of carbonated drinks probably contributes to most of our modern degenerative diseases, obesity and diabetes. To reduce the sugar content, some companies have come up with diet sodas. Unfortunately, as we shall see later, the sugar substitutes used, including aspartame, are even more toxic to our body compared to high sugar itself.

ALKALINE WATER

It has been observed that people and animals living in certain isolated areas of the world seem to have longer age and are more healthy. For years, local people, for instance, those in the Hunza district in Northern Pakistan, believed that it was the water they consumed. There is considerable evidence that this is the case.

The water that falls onto the mountain tops runs through areas of rich mineral deposits. Racing through gravels and waterfalls in a natural process, the result is healthy alkaline water full of useful minerals. This water has been purified by nature without exposure to harmful contaminants and man made chemicals. Due to worldwide environmental pollution and contamination, such natural sources of water are not easily available. Fortunately, we can now achieve the same effect from home based water ionizer.

In a water ionizer, the water is first filtered to remove particulate matter, chlorine and fluorine. This filtered water is then passed into a chamber with platinum electrodes. Alkaline water of up to pH 10 is produced at the cathode while acidic water of pH down to 3 is produced as an effluent.

The alkaline water can be drunk directly and used for making drinks and cooking. The acidic water, on the other hand, can be used for cleaning vegetables, skin and hair. It is a useful antiseptic for superficial wounds. When sprayed on vegetables and plants, it serves to reduce fungal growth and thus encourage plant growth.

The oxidation reduction potential, which is a measure of the antioxidant activity, can be measured at—250mV to—350mV. Furthermore, the electrolysis process reduces the clusters of water from the normal tap water of 11 to 13 to 5 to 7 in alkaline water. Thus alkaline water can penetrate the tissues and organs more effectively, resulting in better rehydration of our body.

There is evidence that alkaline water consumption helps patients with diabetes, high blood pressure and obesity. In fact, water ionizer has been classified as a medical device in Japan for more than ten years.

9

TOXINS

Toxins are chemical substances which interfere with normal chemical processes in the body. In other words, these are poisonous to our body. There are 75,000 chemicals in use today, many of which can cause damage directly or indirectly to our cells.

Pesticides have been implicated in many illnesses, including infertility, cancer, birth defects, skin irritation and impotence. It is estimated that at least 80% of cancers are caused by toxins and carcinogens. While many of these chemicals are easily identified and avoided, many others are hidden in things we consume or use everyday, for instance, shampoos, toothpastes, cosmetics and other products.

CIGARETTE

There is no advantage in smoking except to satisfy addiction in individuals who would otherwise suffer withdrawal symptoms from cessation. How tobacco companies can associate cigarette smoking with healthy living is a good indication of how powerful advertising can influence people's behavior, even when false claims are made.

The hundreds of toxic substances produced from burning tobacco can cause havoc to our lungs, arteries and many other organs, resulting in chronic lung disease, lung cancer, coronary heart disease, cancers of the stomach, intestines etc. Yet it is still extremely difficult to persuade patients to stop smoking. Surely the money could be better spent on more useful activities, quite apart from the money saved from having to seek expensive medical and surgical therapy once any of the diseases strikes.

ENVIRONMENTAL POLLUTION

With increasing industrialization and more widespread usage of motor vehicles, the quality of the air we breathe has obviously deteriorated over the years. These days, even deep sea fish from the North Sea cannot escape from the effects of pollution. Thus, salmon from the North Sea has been found to be contaminated with mercury which is harmful to our brain. This is why pregnant women are advised to limit their consumption of fish.

It was found that people who lived near motorways in Germany developed much higher incidence of all kinds of cancers compared to those who lived far away. The quality of the air can be improved by having trees in the areas we live. These green lungs purify the air. In fact, there is evidence that by placing plants in offices and homes, the quality of air can be improved.

PESTICIDES AND CHEMICAL FERTILIZERS

Modern intensive agricultural methods entail usage of large quantities of pesticides and chemical fertilizers, many of which are toxic to our body. By nature pesticides are chemicals that can kill organisms. How can we assume that we will be immune from them?

Aerial sprays directly pollute our environment. The fungicides and pesticides can affect large areas of the country, carried by weather fronts. Multiple deformities in wild animals, including bony defects, mal-development of organs and premature deaths have been observed. These chemicals can also cause diseases and reactions in human.

Furthermore, these chemicals get into our food chain and our water supply. Many of these are not completely removed before we consume our food or drink our water.

There are alternative ways of agriculture and animal husbandry which would greatly enhance the quality of our food without causing environmental pollution and damage. By definition, organic means produced without the use of pesticides, artificial fertilizers or synthetic chemicals. Whenever possible, organic food would be much preferable to food produced from using large amounts of pesticides and chemical fertilizers. Even though these may be more costly in price, it is well worth paying for our health.

ASPARTAME

This is widely used as a sugar substitute and is promoted for people with diabetes and in diet drinks. In fact, its usage is so widespread that over 5000 food products contain it. Aspartame releases aspartate during digestion. This is an excitatory neurotransmitter. In excess, this can cause death of brain cells and brain tumors.

Aspartame can cause elevated spiking on the EEG (electroencephalogram) resulting in grand mal seizures and blackouts. This is why pilots are advised not to drink too much diet drinks. Aspartame also releases small amount of methanol when broken down in the intestine. Among other effects, methanol causes damage to the retina and optic nerve, resulting in visual problems.

Methanol changes to formaldehyde. This has been implicated in Parkinson's disease, birth defects and Alzheimers disease. Other conditions that have been described include fibromyalgia, leg numbness, vertigo, tinnitus, slurred speech and memory loss. It may be responsible for systemic lupus erythromatosis (SLE) and multiple sclerosis (MS).

Aspartame is thus much more dangerous and harmful than sugar that it was originally designed to replace. How was it that something which could potentially cause so many problems were approved for widespread human consumption? Here again we see the influence of vested interest and big industries. Apparently the original submission for approval was manipulated and at best dubious. However, it has become a multimillion industry with deep pockets. Any attempts to limit its use would be countered by the industry with their own experts counter-arguing and refuting any claims to the contrary.

MONOSODIUM GLUTAMATE

This is used to enhance the taste of food products. It acts as an excitatory neurotransmitter, which is the basis for its usage as a taste enhancer. It also suppresses the undesirable flavors, bitterness and sourness, and eliminates the metallic taste from canned food. Unfortunately, the excitotoxin can cause damage to brain cells by over stimulating them.

The brain is protected to some extent by the blood brain barrier which limits the entry of substances into the brain. The blood brain barrier is not well developed in children. Thus children's brains are four times more sensitive to glutamate induced brain damage than adults. Furthermore, the hypothalamus is not protected by the blood brain barrier. Magnesium and zinc deficiency greatly increases neuronal sensitivity to excitotoxins.

TOXIC CHEMICALS IN COSMETICS AND TOILETRIES

Just pick up any modern shampoo and toothpaste. You may be amazed by the number of synthetic chemicals that are incorporated into each product. Our skin and mucous membrane are good organs of absorption. Long term and repeated exposure may lead to accumulation of these potentially dangerous products.

Sodium lauryl sulphate is widely used in all types of personal care products from liquid soap and shampoo to toothpaste. This is a skin irritant and can cause dermatitis, eczema and psoriasis. It has been shown to slow down tissue healing and may also cause cataract.

The alcohol form of sodium lauryl sulphate is sodium lareth sulphate which is also damaging. The process of ethanolation releases formaldehyde and 1,4 dioxane as contaminants. Another compound called ammonium lauryl sulphate also shows deadly side effects.

Diethanolamine (DEA) is found in shampoo, bubble bath and shaving gel to enhance foaming. This was found to be cancer forming in animals. Parabens—methyl, butyl, ethyl and propyl, are used as preservatives in many products including antiperspirants. These have been linked with breast cancer.

The aluminium in antiperspirants, antacids and antiseptics may have a bearing on Alzheimer's disease, breast cancer and lymphomas. Talc is found in baby powder and other products are found to be toxic. Bentonite, used in cosmetic foundation, may clog pores on skin and lead to skin suffocation.

Collagen, kaolin, mineral oil and petrolatum may all have the same harmful effects on skin. Hair dyes are absorbed through the skin. This has been linked to breast cancer, non-Hodgkins lymphoma. Other toxins that have been identified include mercury, propyl alcohol and plastic products. With environmental pollution, these have been found to contaminate deep sea fish.

10
VITAMINS AND MINERALS

If all our food consists of fresh, organic and natural ingredients full of vitamins and minerals, then perhaps there is no need for any of these supplements. However, modern agricultural methods and food processing have led to a great loss of these essential nutrients. In addition, damaged and thus poisonous materials are daily entering our system from the polluted air we breathe, the contaminated water we drink and the man-made food items devoid of useful nutrients we consume.

The breakdown of our metabolic control resulting in many and varied chronic diseases including diabetes leads to further inability to absorb and utilize vitamins and minerals even when they are present in our food. For these reasons, supplements with vitamins and minerals may be critical in maintaining the well being of some individuals.

Vitamins function as important co-enzymes in various metabolic processes in our body cells. Vitamins were first identified in 1932 when a Polish chemist, Casimir Funk, isolated vitamin B1 from rice. Since then, more than twenty vitamins have been identified.

Deficiency diseases from inadequate vitamin levels in our body have been well described. However, what is not so well known is the subclinical deficiency which may contribute to many degenerative diseases. It is said that anyone who has consumed processed sugar, white flour or canned food has some deficiency disease, the extent of which depending on the proportion of such deprived food in the diet.

Modern food processing destroys many vitamins which occur in natural, optimal proportion for absorption and assimilation in our body. Attempts to enrich such food by adding vitamins may not achieve the desired effects.

Vitamins are divided into two categories. Fat soluble vitamins are vitamins A, D, E and K while water soluble vitamins are vitamins B and C. Fat soluble vitamins require the presence of fat for proper absorption from our gut. People with difficulty absorbing fats, for instance in patients with bile duct obstruction and thus inadequate bile in the intestine, may develop deficiency if prolonged.

Furthermore, modern emphasis on low fat diet may contribute to the deficiency of fat soluble vitamins. Fat soluble vitamins are stored in the body, especially in the liver and fatty tissues such that deficiency states may not develop immediately. On the converse, if excessive fat soluble vitamins are consumed for prolonged periods, toxicity may result from too much accumulation in the body tissues.

Water soluble vitamins are not stored in the body in substantial amounts and thus have to be included in our diet daily. It also means that any excess is excreted in the urine. This is the basis for the idea of expensive urine produced by people who over-consumed vitamins B and C. However, high level of vitamin C in the urine may have beneficial modulating effects on the urinary tract, inhibiting and preventing urinary tract infection and inflammation.

VITAMIN A

The natural form of vitamin A is retinol. The oxidized metabolites, retinaldehyde and retinoic acid are also biologically active. Retinaldehyde is essential for vision while retinoic acid is needed for growth and cell differentiation.

B-carotene is the most common variety in many foods with pro vitamin A activity. Rich sources of vitamin A are found in fish and liver, dark green vegetables and colored fruits. People with vitamin A deficiency may develop difficulty with vision, night blindness and hyperkeratotic skin lesions.

On the other hand, toxicity may result in increased intracranial pressure, vertigo, dry skin, cheilosis, glossitis, alopecia, bone pain, lymph node enlargement. In extreme cases, liver failure may result. High consumption of carotenoids does not result in toxic symptoms but can cause yellowing of skin.

THE B VITAMINS

These are a group of water soluble vitamins which plays important roles in the body's metabolic processes including the metabolism of carbohydrate, fats and sugar. B vitamins are synergistic and are thus more effective when taken together as a group. Thus, B complex vitamins are prepared with many different types of B vitamins. These vitamins are important for the maintenance of muscle tone in stomach and intestine and are good for maintaining the health of skin, hair, eyes, mouth and liver.

VITAMIN B1—THIAMINE

Thiamine was the first vitamin isolated. It is important for energy production and carbohydrate metabolism. Thiamine combines with pyruvic acid to form energy. It acts as the co-enzyme for the production of acetylcholine.

Thiamine is also a powerful antioxidant. Thus, thiamine is important for promoting growth. Dietary sources of thiamine include yeast, pork, legumes, beef, whole grains and nut. Polished white rice unfortunately contains little thiamine. Thiamine is also heat sensitive.

The requirement for vitamin B1 increases during illness, stress and surgery. Thus deficiency may result in people with poor dietary intake, alcoholics and patients with chronic diseases including cancer. This results in anorexia, irritability, apathy and generalized weakness.

In prolonged cases, beriberi may result, with features of enlarged heart, peripheral edema, peripheral neuritis. In dry beriberi, symmetrical peripheral neuropathy of the motor and sensory nerves and diminished reflexes may result. Patients taking diuretic tablets tend to lose more thiamine. Hemodialysis also leads to increased loss.

VITAMIN B2—RIBOFLAVIN

This vitamin is essential for the metabolism of fat, carbohydrate and protein. It aids in growth and reproduction, promotes healthy skin, nail and hair, helps in reducing sore mouth, lips and tongue and alleviates eye fatigue. It is an antioxidant and it protects the body against free radicals. Dietary sources are milk, meat, egg, broccoli and legumes. Deficiency may result in mucocutaneous lesions, skin abnormalities and corneal vascularization.

VITAMIN B3—NIACIN

This is important for fatty acid synthesis and protein metabolism. It is needed for the maintenance of healthy skin, nerves and gastrointestinal tract. Niacin has been shown to reduce low density lipoprotein cholesterol and increase high density lipoprotein cholesterol. Niacin is found in protein rich food such as meats, fish, yeast, legumes and nuts. Deficiency results in pellagra, loss of appetite, general weakness, abdominal pain and vomiting.

VITAMIN B5—PANTOTHENIC ACID

Pantothenic acid is important for the conversion of fat and sugar into energy. It is used for the synthesis of coenzyme A for biochemical reactions and functions as a coenzyme in carboxylation reactions.

It is vital for adrenal function and antibody production. It aids in wound healing. It prevents fatigue. Pantothenic acid is produced by bacteria in our intestines. Rich sources are found in meats, legumes and whole grain cereals.

VITAMIN B 6-PYRIDOXINE

Pyridoxine is important for amino acid metabolism, heme and neurotransmitter synthesis. This is essential for the synthesis of antibodies and right blood cells and is required for the absorption of vitamin B12. Dietary sources include legumes, nuts, wheat germ, cabbage, eggs, beef.

Deficiency results in seborrheic dermatitis, glossitis, stomatitis and cheilosis. It may also result in general weakness, peripheral neuropathy and hyperhomocystinemia. The requirement for vitamin B6 is increased when high protein diets are consumed. Vitamin B6 helps prevent various nervous and skin diseases. It relieves nausea and is used for morning sickness from pregnancy. It promotes the synthesis of anti-aging nucleic acid, helps reduce dry mouth and works as a natural diuretic. Vitamin B6 reduces the requirement for insulin in diabetics.

VITAMIN B9—FOLIC ACID

This interacts with vitamin B12 and is important for DNA synthesis. It is essential for hemoglobin and right blood cell formation. It is also important for protein, amino acid and sugar metabolism. A deficiency of folic acid causes anemia, poor growth and irritation of the skin.

The need for folic acid increases during pregnancy and lactation. The daily recommended allowance for folic acid is 400 mcg. This is double in pregnancy. Heavy drinker also needs to increase folic acid intake. Large doses of vitamin C increases urinary excretion of folic acid. Dietary sources include liver, yeast, and green vegetables.

Folic acid improves lactation and may protect against food poisoning. It promotes healthy skin, delays hair graying and improves appetite. It may also provide pain relief. Folate is essential for the repair and replication of DNA. Folate deficiency plays a part in many types of cancer, including colon cancer, rectal cancers, breast cancer, pancreatic and brain cancer.

Folate, vitamin B6 and vitamin B12 reduce the levels of homocysteine, which plays a crucial role in heart disease. In fact, homocysteine levels correlate much better than the levels of cholesterol in patients with heart disease. There is also a link between folate deficiency and depression. Adequate level of folate can also reduce the risk of Alzheimer's disease.

VITAMIN B12—COBALAMINE

Vitamin B12 is necessary for the metabolism of carbohydrates, proteins and fats. This is essential for the formation and regeneration of red blood cells. Vitamin B12 is required for the formation of nerve sheaths. It promotes growth and improves appetite in children. It is important for maintaining a healthy nervous system.

Vitamin B12 absorption depends on the availability of intrinsic factor from the stomach. Thus patients who had part of their stomach removed may have difficulty absorbing sufficient vitamin B12. They may then develop pernicious anemia which causes weakness, numbness, pallor, fever and other symptoms. These patients may require regular injections of vitamin B12 for optimal health. Rich sources of vitamin B12 include egg yolk, poultry and milk. Vitamin B12 is not found in plant food sources.

VITAMIN B13—OROTIC ACID

This is important for the metabolism of folic acid and vitamin B12. It prevents alcoholic liver problems and premature aging. It may help in multiple sclerosis. It is found in root vegetables and whey.

VITAMIN B15—PANGAMIC ACID

This is an antioxidant and may extend cell life span. It may reduce the craving for alcoholic liquor and lower blood cholesterol. It may protect against pollution and relieve the symptoms of angina and asthma. It also stimulates immune responses.

INOSITOL

This combines with choline to form lecithin and is important for brain function. It is important for the metabolism of fats and cholesterol. It promotes healthy hair and reduces eczema. It helps lower cholesterol levels. Dietary sources are liver, yeast, dried lima beans, cantaloupe, grapefruit, raisins, peanuts, cabbage. Heavy coffee drinkers may need supplemental inositol.

CHOLINE

This is another B family vitamin. It is important for fat and cholesterol utilization. It emulsifies cholesterol so that it doesn't settle on artery walls or in the gallbladder to form gallstones. Choline can penetrate the blood brain barrier and may aid memory. It aids in the transmission of nerve impulses, especially those associated with the formation of memory.

It helps to eliminate poisons and drugs by aiding the liver. It may help in the treatment of Alzheimer's disease. Deficiency may result in cirrhosis, fatty liver, hardening of the arteries and Alzheimer's disease. Dietary sources include egg yolk, heart, green leafy vegetables, yeast, liver and wheat germ.

PABA—PARA-AMINOBENZOIC ACID

This can be synthesized in the body. It helps form folic acid and is important in the utilization of protein. It helps in the assimilation of pantothenic acid. It has sun-screening properties. Thus, used as an ointment it can protect against sunburn. It reduces the pain of burns. It helps to delay wrinkles and keep skin healthy. It may restore natural color to the hair. Dietary sources include liver, yeast, kidney, whole grains, rice, bran and wheat germ. Penicillin and sulpha drugs increase the need for PABA.

VITAMIN C—ASCORBIC ACID

Vitamin C has wide ranging effects in the body. It is required for collagen synthesis. It is a strong antioxidant protecting against free radicals, pollution, carcinogens, heavy metals and other toxins. It has strong antiviral and mild antibacterial properties. It also acts to regenerate other antioxidants such as vitamin E and glutathione.

It is present in high concentration in adrenal glands and is essential for the synthesis of stress hormones and aldosterone. Vitamin C is essential for both cellular and humoral immunity. Energy cannot be made in any cell without adequate vitamin C.

It is important for the conversion of dopamine to noradrenaline. It is an important component of many drug metabolizing enzymes. Dietary sources include citrus fruits, green vegetables especially broccoli, tomatoes and potatoes. Smoking, hemodialysis, stress, pregnancy, lactation increase vitamin C requirement. Each cigarette can destroy 25 to 100 mg of vitamin C.

Vitamin C is so central in so many chemical reactions in the body that life is not possible without it. Unlike other vitamins, vitamin C is required in large amounts which could only be supplied by a diet high in fruit and vegetables. All mammals, with the exception of guinea pigs, fruit eating bats and primates including man make their own vitamin C from glucose.

The daily requirement for a man is probably in the region of 3 g to 15 g, with an average of 5.4 g. Under conditions of stress or infection, the requirement may quadruple. The recommended daily dosage of 60 mg may be sufficient to prevent scurvy but is probably far inadequate in patients with acute and chronic illnesses.

Large doses of vitamin C have been successfully used to treat common cold and other viral infections. To be successful, vitamin C treatment must be intensive. Vitamin C appears to remove the protective protein coat of the virus thus killing them. Herpes zoster, herpes simplex, adenovirus, measles and other viruses all appear to be susceptible to vitamin C.

Vitamin C also strengthens humoral and cellular immune systems and thus resistance to the viruses. The role of vitamin C in eliminating viral infection may have a bearing on certain cancers including cancer of the cervix, breast and lymphoma. Vitamin C may prevent the recurrence of bladder cancer. Cancer patients require large doses of vitamin C to prolong their survival. Vitamin C may enable larger and more prolonged doses of radiation therapy to be carried out. It will also prevent radiation injury to tissues.

Large doses of vitamin C may relieve the symptoms of urethritis. In pregnancy, the requirement for vitamin C is increased. Intravenous vitamin C injection may reduce intraocular pressure to improve glaucoma. Vitamin C can also reduce the pressure of intervertebral disc in cases of disc herniation.

Vitamin C can protect against lead and mercury poisoning. Also, carbon monoxide poisoning can be averted by large doses of vitamin C. Some city dwellers are frequently exposed to 100 ppm of carbon monoxide that may lead to carboxyhemoglobin level of up to 10%. This may have profound depressing effect on cardiac function.

One theory of atherosclerosis proposes that relative lack of vitamin C leads to collagen weakness and thus damage to vessel walls which then lead to the formation of atherosclerotic plagues. In animals, high doses of vitamin C have been shown to reverse these plagues. Vitamin C reduces cholesterol level in the blood. The strengthening effect on the collagen further contributes to the increased strength and elasticity of the blood vessels.

Another theory implies infection, either viral or bacterial, as playing a part in the initiation of atherosclerosis. Here as well, the beneficial effects of vitamin C may be present.

Linus Pauling, who was awarded two Nobel prizes, for chemistry and medicine, proposed the unified theory for heart disease as a manifestation of chronic vitamin C deficiency. Since collagen is the most abundant protein in the body and is vitally important for the strength and elasticity of blood vessels and since vitamin C is essential for the synthesis of collagen, vitamin C deficiency leads to weakened blood vessel walls.

These occur at areas of turbulence which corresponds to the places prone to develop atherosclerosis. Thus, cracks and mini breaks occur at these places, leading to deposition of cholesterol and calcium in order to strengthen these areas. Lipoprotein a is the initiator of this event and its levels have been well correlated with the development of coronary heart disease.

Vitamin C supplementation, in adequate doses (3-6 g per day) strengthens the collagen and blood vessel walls, and has been demonstrated to lower the level of lipoprotein a. This may lead to a reversal of atherosclerosis and a cure for heart disease.

VITAMIN D—CALCIFEROL

Vitamin D is essential for calcium and phosphorus metabolism. This vitamin can be made in the skin from cholesterol precursor on exposure to sunlight. However, in places where sunlight exposure is inadequate, supplements may be necessary. Dietary sources include fish liver oils, sardines, herring, salmon, milk and dairy products.

The recommended daily requirement is 200 IU per day up to 50 years, 400 to 600 IU per day for older people. Deficiency causes rickets and osteoporosis. Since this is fat soluble, excessive intake may lead to toxicity which may manifest as unusual thirst, sore eyes, itchy skin, vomiting, abnormal calcium deposits in blood vessel wall, liver, lungs, kidney and stomach.

VITAMIN E—TOCOPHEROL

There are eight naturally occurring plant compounds with vitamin E activity. Alpha tocopherol is the most active. Vitamin E is an effective antioxidant and it inhibits prostaglandin synthesis. Dietary sources include wheat germ, vegetable oils, green vegetables, whole grain cereals and eggs.

Unlike other fat soluble vitamins, vitamin E is stored in the body for a relatively short time, much of it being excreted in the feces. Vitamin E helps to supply oxygen to the body and may protect the lungs against air pollution. It prevents and dissolves blood clots, prevents thick scar formation and miscarriages. It may also help leg cramps.

Vitamin E deficiency causes red blood cell destruction, muscle degeneration and reproductive disorders. The recommended daily dose is 8 to 10 IU. Large doses (>800 IU) may lead to spontaneous hemorrhage from inhibition of platelet aggregation. Vitamin E may interfere with anticoagulation and anti-platelet therapy and it contraindicated in patients taking Coumadin.

VITAMIN K

There are two natural forms of vitamin K, phylloquinone from vegetables and animal sources and menaquinone which is synthesised by natural bacteria in the intestine. Vitamin K is essential for the formation of prothrombin needed for blood clotting. Thus, vitamin K helps in preventing internal bleeding and reduces menstrual flow. Dietary sources include yoghurt, egg yolk, fish liver oil, kelp, green leafy vegetables. Deficiency may lead to hemorrhage. Vitamin K interferes with Coumadin therapy and should not be taken by patients on this medication.

Apart from clotting, vitamin K is also essential for strong bones and prevention of heart disease. Vitamin K improves bone density and prevents osteoporosis. It may help to keep calcium out of arterial linings and thus prevent heart disease. Vitamin K may also help to fight cancer, including lung cancer. Vitamin K deficiency may contribute to Alzheimer's disease and interfere with insulin release.

MINERALS

CALCIUM

Calcium is the most abundant mineral in the body, forming 1 to 2 kg in adults. Most of the body's calcium is in the bones and teeth. Twenty percent of the adult's bone calcium is reabsorbed and replaced every year. Calcium and phosphorus work together for healthy bones and teeth. Together with magnesium, it is important for cardiovascular health.

In order for calcium to be absorbed, there must be sufficient vitamin D. The recommended daily allowance for adults is between 800 to 1200 mg. Calcium helps to metabolize iron. Dietary sources of calcium include milk, cheese, soybeans, peanuts, walnuts, sunflower seeds and green vegetables. Calcium deficiency results in rickets, osteomalacia and osteoporosis. Large quantities of fat, oxalic acid in chocolate and rhubard and phytic acid in grains may prevent calcium absorption.

CHROMIUM

Chromium works with insulin in sugar metabolism. It potentiates the action of insulin. It aids growth and helps prevent and lower blood pressure. Chromium deficiency may be a factor in arteriosclerosis and diabetes. Dietary sources include meat, shellfish, chicken, clams, yeast.

COBALT

This is part of vitamin B12 and is essential for red blood cell formation. The dietary sources are meat, kidney, liver, milk, oysters and clams. Strict vegetarian may be deficient in cobalt, resulting in anemia.

COPPER

Copper is an integral part of many enzyme systems. Copper plays an important part in iron metabolism, melanin synthesis, central nervous system function and the synthesis of elastin and collagen. It is essential for the utilization of vitamin C. The daily recommended allowance is 1.5 to 3 mg. Rich sources are found in shellfish, liver, nuts, legumes and meats. Deficiency causes anemia and edema.

IRON

Iron is absolutely required for life. It is required for the synthesis of hemoglobin, myoglobin and many enzymes. Only about 8 percent of the total iron intake is absorbed. The daily recommended allowance is 10 to 18 mg for adults, 30 to 60 mg for pregnant and lactating women. Copper, cobalt, manganese and vitamin C are necessary to assimilate iron.

Iron is necessary for the proper utilization of B vitamins. Iron aids growth, increases resistance to disease, prevents fatigue and improves skin tone. Dietary sources include liver, kidney, heart, red meat, egg yolks, oysters, nuts, beans, asparagus and oatmeal. Deficiency results in anemia. Inorganic iron, ferrous sulphate, can destroy vitamin E whereas organic iron including ferrous gluconate, fumarate, citrate and peptonate do not. Heavy drinkers of coffee and tea may have insufficient absorption of iron.

MAGNESIUM

Magnesium is needed for the metabolism of calcium, vitamin C, phosphorus, sodium and potassium. It is essential for nerve and muscle functioning. It is important for converting blood sugar into energy. Adults need 300 to 450 mg daily.

The human body contains about 20 g of magnesium. Magnesium promotes a healthy cardiovascular system and helps prevent heart attacks. It helps prevent calcium deposits, kidney stones and gallstones. It relieves indigestion and keeps teeth healthy. Dietary sources include figs, lemons, grapefruit, corn, almonds, nuts, dark green vegetables and apples. Alcoholics may be deficient in magnesium. Women on the pill or hormone replacement therapy may need magnesium supplement.

MANGANESE

Manganese helps to activate enzymes necessary for the proper usage of biotin, thiamine and vitamin C. It is needed for normal bone structure. It is also important for the formation of thyroxine, digestion and utilisation of food. Manganese is important for reproduction and central nervous system function. It can help fatigue and improve memory. Deficiency causes ataxia. Dietary sources include nuts, green vegetables, peas, egg yolks and whole grain cereals.

ZINC

Zinc is essential for protein synthesis, insulin formation, muscle contraction and maintenance of acid-base balance. It exerts a normalizing effect on the prostate and is important in the reproductive system. The daily recommended allowance is 15 mg for adults.

Most zinc in food is lost in processing. Zinc accelerates healing for wounds, improves taste, promotes growth and mental alertness. It may reduce cholesterol deposits. Deficiency may result in prostate hypertrophy and arteriosclerosis. Dietary sources are steak, lamb chops, pork loin, wheat germ, yeast, pumpkin seeds, eggs, ground mustard. Alcoholics and diabetics need higher intake of zinc.

MOLYBDENUM

Molybdenum is a vital part of the enzyme for iron utilization. It is important for carbohydrate and fat metabolism. Molybdenum helps to prevent anemia and promotes general well being. Dietary sources are dark green vegetables, whole grains and legumes. Deficiency is rare.

PHOSPHORUS

Phosphorus is present in every cell in the body. Vitamin D and calcium are needed for phosphorus functioning. Phosphorus is involved in virtually all physiological chemical reactions. It is necessary for normal bone and tooth structure, heart regularity, kidney function and nerve impulse transmission. The daily recommended dose is 800 to 1200 mg for adults.

Phosphorus helps in growth and body repair, promotes healthy gums and teeth, and lessens the arthritic pain. Deficiency results in rickets. Dietary sources include fish, poultry, meat, whole grains, eggs, nuts, seeds. Too much phosphorus upsets mineral balance and decreases calcium.

POTASSIUM

Potassium is the commonest intracellular cation. It works with sodium to regulate the body's water balance. It is important for maintaining heart rhythm, nerve and muscle functions. Hypoglycemia and diarrhea cause potassium loss. Potassium helps to reduce blood pressure and allergy. Dietary sources include citrus fruits, cantaloupe, tomatoes, watercress, green leafy vegetables, mint leaves, sunflower seeds, bananas and potatoes. A dosage of 25 g of potassium chloride can cause toxicity. Heavy coffee drinkers may develop low potassium, so can heavy drinkers and high sugar intake.

SELENIUM

Selenium has a synergistic effect with vitamin E. It is an antioxidant. Men need more selenium since the male reproductive tract contains high concentration of it. Selenium is lost in the semen. Selenium aids in keeping elasticity in tissues, alleviates hot flashes and menopausal symptoms. It helps in the treatment and prevention of dandruff and may neutralize carcinogens and provide protection from some cancers. Dietary sources include wheat germ, bran, tuna, onions, tomatoes and broccoli.

SODIUM

Sodium is essential for normal growth. High intake of sodium results in potassium depletion and high blood pressure. It is important for nerve conduction and muscle function. Deficiency results in impaired carbohydrate digestion and neuralgia. Dietary sources include salt, shellfish, carrots, beets, artichokes, kidney, bacon and kelp.

SULPHUR

Sulphur is essential for healthy hair, skin and nails. It helps maintain oxygen balance and amino acid metabolism. It helps the liver to secrete bile and helps fight bacterial infections. Dietary sources include beef, beans, fish, eggs and cabbage. Sulphur creams and ointments have been used to treat a variety of skin problems.

IODINE

Iodine is essential for thyroid hormone formation. Two thirds of the body's iodine are concentrated in the thyroid gland. Iodine promotes proper growth, improves energy, burns excess fat, improves mental alacrity and healthy hair, nails, skin and teeth. Deficiency results in hypothyroidism and goitre. Dietary sources include kelp, onions, all seafoods. Raw cabbage prevents proper utilization of iodine. Iodine has useful wide spectrum antiseptic properties not only for superficial skin infections but also for respiratory and other infections.

JUICING FOR HEALTH

Most of the vitamins and minerals essential for our health and wellbeing can be found in fruits and vegetables. Our body does not have the necessary enzyme to digest cellulose in the plant cell wall. Thus, many of the useful ingredients eaten in salads are not adequately absorbed. This may help our intestinal health by increasing the bulk of our stools, but it may not provide sufficient micronutrients important for our cellular wellbeing. Cooking breaks down some of the barriers. Unfortunately cooking also destroys some of the micronutrients.

The best way to obtain vitamins and minerals from fruits and vegetables is probably by juicing. By using sensible combinations, not only can the juice provide ideal micronutrients, but also the taste can be enhanced. A useful combination is using celery, cucumber, green pepper, bitter gourd and green apple.

Freshly made juices are full of healthy micronutrients. It is desirable to consume these as soon as they are made. The quality deteriorates with time. Thus, preserved juices, even though they are claimed to be totally natural, are not as good. Since juicers are easily available and cheap, and fruits and vegetables are usually abundant in most countries, juicing should be encouraged. Of course, if you are able to obtain good organic fruits and vegetables, that would be ideal.

11

NATURAL HEALING

Until the advent of modern pharmaceutical procedures in synthesizing drugs, man relied on natural substances to overcome illnesses and to strengthen their body against infections and other diseases. In many cultures, there still exist many tried and tested natural therapies. In fact, the earlier medicinal products were extracted from plants. Knowledge of these natural healing methods may enhance our well being without doing any harm to our body during the process.

Our body needs an adequate intake of protein in order to repair damaged parts and to regenerate others. There are eight essential amino acids, the building blocks for protein which cannot be made in our body and thus have to be taken in sufficient amount in our diet. These, apart from forming part of the structural proteins in our body, may also have additional properties which double their importance for our health and well being. The essential amino acids are leucine, lysine, methionine, phenylalanine, threonine, tryptophan, valine and isoleucine.

TRYPTOPHAN

Tryptophan is essential for the production of serotonin, a neurotransmitter involved in sleep. Thus, tryptophan helps to induce sleep. It also reduces pain sensitivity, has an antidepressant effect and reduces anxiety and tension. It is found in cottage cheese, milk, meat, turkey, bananas, dates and peanuts.

PHENYLALANINE

This can act as a neurotransmitter. It is converted into noradrenaline and dopamine in the adrenal gland. It can reduce hunger and improve sexual drive. It may improve memory and alertness and alleviate depression. It is found in abundance in protein rich foods, almonds, lima beans, pumpkin and sesame seeds.

LYSINE

This is essential for tissue repair, growth, production of antibodies, hormones and enzymes. It alleviates herpes simplex infection and improves mental concentration. It also helps in some fertility problems.

ARGININE

Arginine is required for the synthesis and release of growth hormone. The seminal fluid contains high concentration of arginine. It increases sperm count, improves immune response and wound healing. It also helps to metabolize stored fat and tone up muscles.

ORNITHINE

Ornithine stimulates insulin secretion. It helps insulin work as anabolic hormone to increase fat and energy storage.

GLUTAMIC ACID AND GLUTAMINE

Glutamic acid is brain fuel. In the presence of ammonia, our body converts it into glutamine. Glutamine appears to improve intelligence and control alcoholism. It improves ulcer healing and alleviates fatigue, depression and impotence.

ASPARTIC ACID

Aspartic acid aids in the expulsion of harmful ammonia from the body. It thus protects the brain.

CYSTINE AND CYSTEINE

Cystine is the stable form of the sulphur containing amino acid. They have strong antioxidant properties.

METHIONINE

Methionine helps in pituitary function. It is useful in progressive muscular dystrophy, hypoglycaemia and schizophrenia.

TYROSINE

This acts as a neurotranstter. It helps depression.

GLUTATHIONE

L-glutathione is a tripeptide made up of L-cysteine, L-glutamic acid and glycine. Glutathione is the most abundant and most important antioxidant in the body. Without proper level of glutathione, cells undergo programmed cell death (apoptosis). Glutathione levels in cells are influenced by vitamin B6, Riboflavin, copper and selenium. Glutathione recharges vitamins C and E to be reused.

Glutathione deficiency is linked to mitochondrial dysfunction and thus ATP (adenosine triphosphate) synthesis. The energy available to do work in the cells is equivalent to the glutathione concentration. Glutathione also potentiates the action of insulin and improves natural killer cell activity. Glutathione supports the immune system and helps the liver to detoxify toxins. Low levels of glutathione are found in cancer, Parkinson's disease, Alzheimers disease, diabetes, artherosclerosis, hepatitis, multiple sclerosis, AIDS. Its level also decreases with aging. Glutathione prevents the harmful effects of high dose radiation and protects against cigarette smoke and alcohol. It is useful for emphysema.

GRAPE SEED EXTRACT

For years the French had lower incidence of coronary heart disease. One of the factors proposed for this was the consumption of red wine. More recently, it was found that the oligomeric proanthocyanidins (OPC's) were a group of compounds found in red wine which had strong antioxidant effect on the body. In fact, it was the grape derivative which serves this role rather than the alcohol content of the red wine.

OPC's are found in abundance in red grapes, especially in the skin and the seed. In fact, grape seeds have the highest concentration of the useful OPC's. Grape seed extract has been used in numerous settings. It strong antioxidant effect is particularly beneficial in degenerative diseases including coronary heart disease, and may have anticarcinogenic effects. OPC's have potent effect on collagen and thus strengthen capillaries and enhance blood flow in the veins.

The antioxidant effect is claimed to be fifty times more potent than vitamin E and twenty times more potent than vitamin C. By improving endothelial function, OPC's may prevent the initiation of atherosclerosis. Furthermore, OPC's decrease lipid peroxidation and oxidation of LDL cholesterol. This beneficial effect was measured using brachial artery reactivity testing.

OPC's decreases platelet aggregation and thus thrombosis. This protects against acute heart attack. They also increase the level of nitric oxide. OPC's increase natural killer cell activity and antimutagenicity. OPC's promote hair growth and encourage the proliferation of hair follicle cells. OPC's can cross the blood brain membrane and thus may have beneficial effects on brain protection. This may be useful for treating multiple sclerosis. As for the eyes, OPC's slow down macular degeneration and cataract. They slow down some retinopathy.

GRAPEFRUIT SEED EXTRACT

Grapefruit seed extract has been found to be antibacterial and also effective against viruses, yeast, fungi and parasites. It contains many polyphenolic compounds which are converted into quaternary ammonium compounds which have broad spectrum antimicrobial activity. Grape fruit extract inhibits the enzymes responsible for maintaining microbial cell membrane, leading to the loss of the cytoplasmic membrane. It can also be used to protect fish and poultry against Salmonella and E. Coli infections.

Grapefruit seed extract is used as disinfectant and sanitizing agent for many hospitals in the United States. At higher concentration, it is used for sterilizing and disinfecting operation rooms. Added to inhalers, this is useful for the control of respiratory infections.

OLIVE LEAF EXTRACT

Olive leaf extract contains oleuropein which has antibacterial and antioxidant properties. This has been shown to cause relaxation of arterial wall in animals and may be useful for treating hypertension. It also lowers blood sugar and uric acid levels. It also stops viral replication by interfering with amino acid synthesis.

By interfering with the production of reverse transcriptase, it inhibits retroviruses and thus may be useful against AIDS. In mouse phagocytes, olive leaf extract was shown to increase nitric oxide production and thus phagocytosis. It protects LDL cholesterol from oxidation and may have a beneficial effect on atherosclerosis.

CRANBERRY EXTRACT

As previously discussed in the section on sugars, cranberry extract contains D-mannose, which prevents the adhesions of E.Coli to the urogenital tract and thus is useful for treating urinary tract infections. It is also a useful antioxidant and has been shown to reduce the damage from stroke.

COLOSTRUM

Colostrum milk is the first milk secreted by lactating mothers. As such, it contains many useful substances which play a vital role in the development of the immune system in the young. Bovine colostrum contains more than 250 substances which are potentially beneficial to health. There are numerous immune factors, growth factors, vitamins, minerals and amino acids.

In fact, bovine colostrum has forty times more immune factors than human colostrum. Lactoferrin in colostrum binds iron. Colostrum may also detoxify lead. Colostrum is a useful supplement for general well being of the body and may be useful against bacterial infections including sinusitis, bronchitis and urinary infection.

BEE PRODUCTS

Many items derived from honey bees have beneficial effects to our health. Honey is a good source of energy and is rich in B vitamins, vitamins C, D and E and trace elements. It also has useful antibacterial properties against salmonella, E.Coli, shigella and candida. Used as dressing, honey is useful in treating burns and wounds.

Bee pollen is 35% protein. It contains fatty acids and lecithin, vitamins B and C, and minerals including iron, zinc, magnesium, calcium, copper and selenium. It is rich in phytochemicals including carotenoids, flavonoids and phytosterols. It may reduce tumor growth, reduce enlarged prostate and prostatitis, improve skin elasticity and reduce wrinkles.

Propolis has strong antibacterial, antiviral and antifungal properties. It contains many flavonoids. It strengthens the immune system, reduces dental plaque and caries and may reduce the pain of herpes. It is also effective against staphlococcus aureus.

Royal jelly has strong antibacterial properties. It is rich in vitamins, amino acids and minerals. It helps wounds to heal and may have anticancer properties.

EVENING PRIMROSE OIL

Evening primrose oil contains rich gamma linolenic acid (GLA), an essential fatty acid needed for prostaglandin systhesis. This controls cell growth, maturation cycle and blood pressure. GLA has been shown to reduce the symptoms of post-menapausal syndrome and arthritis. It has antioxidant properties. GLA increases sex hormone synthesis, including estrogen and testosterone. It reduces cholesterol level and may be useful for cirrhosis.

FLAXSEED

Ground flaxseeds are rich in omega 3 fatty acid, lignans, fibre and contain high levels of protein, B vitamins, vitamin E and minerals including selenium, calcium, potassium, magnesium, manganese and zinc. Flaxseed oil has been found to have anticancer properties and also prevent heart disease. A combination of flaxseed oil and cottage cheese forms the basis of the Budwig diet for cancer.

BUCKWHEAT

Buckwheat contains 31% more protein than brown rice and 43% more protein than polished rice. Buckwheat is rich in flavonoids especially rutin which has antioxidant properties. It protects LDL cholesterol from oxidation and strengthens capillaries.

Buckwheat is rich in magnesium which relaxes blood vessels and improves blood flow. This may be beneficial in reducing blood pressure. Buckwheat has been found to be good for diabetes. It is able to reduce glucose by 12 to 19% due to its higher concentration of protein.

BILBERRY

Bilberry extract contains high levels of tannic acid, cinnamic acid, flavonols, anthocyanidins and isoflavones. It has been found useful in diseases of the eyes including retinitis pigmentosa, diabetic and hypertensive retinopathy, retinal inflammation, macular degeneration, glaucoma, cataract and night vision. The anthocyanidins protect and regulate rhodopsin which is essential for central vision in the macula.

Age related macular degeneration is now the leading cause of blindness in the western world. Bilberry extract has been found to prevent and also to reverse some of the changes of macular degeneration. The anthocyanidins also reduce blood pressure, blood clotting and improves blood supply. By reducing vascular permeability, it reduces the exudate which forms in the wet form of macular degeneration.

SAW PALMETTO

This is the extract from the berries of a small palm tree. It contains free fatty acids, phytosterols and monoglycerides. It has long been used to improve urinary flow in people with prostate hypertrophy. Saw palmetto blocks the production of dihydrotesterone which helps in reducing benign prostatic hypertrophy. The antioxidant and anti-inflammatory effects may be useful in other areas including improving lactation, libido, hair growth and thyroid deficiency.

ALMOND

Almond contains high quality protein, monounsaturated fatty acids, dietary fibre, alpha-tocopherol and is also rich in magnesium, calcium, potassium, copper, manganese and phosphorus. It also have high flavonoids which have useful anti-oxidant effects. It has been shown to reduce blood sugar level and the level of low density lipoprotein. It also increases the level of high density lipoprotein and thus may protect the heart against coronary artery disease. It is useful for anemia, bone mass and eczema.

ACAI

This little berry from the Amazon jungle is packed with nutrients. It contains ten times the antioxidants of grapes. Its vitamin C content is 65 times that of oranges. Its high content of phytosterols, flavonoids and essential fatty acids makes it one of nature's healthiest fruits for consumption.

12

EXERCISE

Physical exercise has numerous benefits. Regular exercise enables more people to live longer and better. Combined with attention to diet and avoidance of toxins, exercise will improve the sense of well being and reduce the risk of depression and anxiety. Exercise improves heart function by increasing the efficiency of the heart muscle. Muscular strength in general is also strengthened. This leads to improved mobility, flexibility and balance, especially in older people.

Exercise improves lung capacity and blood supply to tissues and organs. It also improves bone strength, reduces body fat and increases lean body tissue. It reduces the risk of osteoporosis. Regular exercise improves blood sugar control and insulin resistance and is thus vital for diabetic patients. It also leads to a reduction in blood pressure, reduced triglyceride levels and improved high density lipoprotein cholesterol, all of which may help in cardiovascular diseases. Regular exercise is a must for weight management in people with any degree of obesity.

TYPES OF EXERCISE

Aerobic exercise provides a foundation for physical fitness. It involves a large number of muscle groups used for at least twenty minutes in order to derive cardiovascular benefits. It also improves lung function. Walking is a good form of exercise, so is jogging, running, aerobic dance, bicycling, rowing, swimming and cross country skiing.

Resistance training involves work against gravity. Weight lifting is a form of resistance training, as is push up and climbing. Resistance training may be even more important in older people since it helps to preserve bone and muscle mass, an effect which can be achieved more than with aerobic exercises. Flexibility and balance training improve coordination and may reduce falls in the elderly.

Within these groups, there are so many different types of exercise that can be done. It is important to choose something which you like to do. Having a partner to share the exercise would also help. It is important to start slowly, especially for somebody unaccustomed to heavy physical exercise. People with heart and other diseases should undergo a full medical assessment prior to strenuous exercise. Certainly if moderate exercise induces chest or jaw pain, breathlessness and dizziness, then great caution has to be taken. However, even patients with established heart and other diseases can benefit from some form of exercise.

Probably the easiest, cheapest and safest form of exercise is walking. Brisk walking probably benefits more than leisurely stroll. Young and fit people could push themselves to the brink without any harm. However, older people and those with various diseases may be harm by too strenuous an activity. The general guideline is to walk at a pace which allows conversation to continue and without breathlessness.

A more scientific check is to monitor the heart rate during exercise. The maximal achievable heart rate can be estimated by subtracting the age from 220. The target is to achieve a heart rate of 50% to 75% of the maximal heart rate. The heart rate can be counted by light pressure on the radial artery at the wrist. Count for 15 seconds and multiply by 4. Wrist worn electronic devices are available which would give instant heart rate reading.

Walking is thus a good form of physical exercise for all ages. Brisk walking provides strenuous enough exercise for cardiovascular training in most adults. Unlike running, walking puts little strain on knees and legs. A long term program of walking may increase longevity. Walking has to be done for at least 30 minutes to provide cardiovascular benefits. There is evidence that even breaking the thirty minutes into ten minute blocks achieves the same result.

Physical exercise can be incorporated into most people's daily routine. Thus, instead of taking the elevators, walking up stairs would be more useful. Parking the car some distance away and walking to the place of work or shopping mall, gardening, even washing the car can all contribute to the physical exercise that can be accumulated throughout the day.

EXERCISE AND HEART DISEASE

Regular physical exercise may reduce the risk of heart disease by up to 40%. This is achieved by the beneficial effects on the heart function, reduction of blood pressure, decrease in triglyceride level and an increase in the high density lipoprotein (HDL) level. An improvement in glucose metabolism and insulin resistance also helps to reduce the risk of cardiovascular deaths in people with diabetes.

Inactive people are at the highest risk of heart disease. Since the heart is a muscular pump, physical exercise conditions the heart and makes it pump stronger. A strong, well-conditioned heart pumps the same amount of blood in 50 beats as the weaker heart pumping for 75 beats. At rest, a well conditioned heart in a fit, athletic individual beats at a slow rate.

EXERCISE AND MENTAL HEALTH

Regular physical activity has a positive effect on our well being and mental health. Exercises reduce anxiety and depression. They also improve self esteem. Regular physical activity improves our sleep pattern and the quality of our sleep. Morning exercise appears to have a more beneficial effect on our sleep pattern rather than exercise later in the day due to the hormonal changes which accompany physical exertion.

EXERCISE AND CANCER

Regular exercise can reduce the risk of cancer. Colonic cancer can be reduced by up to 40% with a program of regular physical exercise. This is achieved by increased bowel movement, change in insulin resistance, hormonal, inflammatory and immunological factors. The same rate of reduction is also seen in breast cancer in both pre and post menopausal women. Prostate cancer is 10% less in people who are physically active. The beneficial effects of exercise on sex hormones lead to a 30% reduction in endometrial cancer. Lung cancer rate can also be reduced by 30 to 40% by regular physical exercise.

978-0-595-36432-
0-595-36432-2